I0813869

HOSPITALS

by Emma Bassier

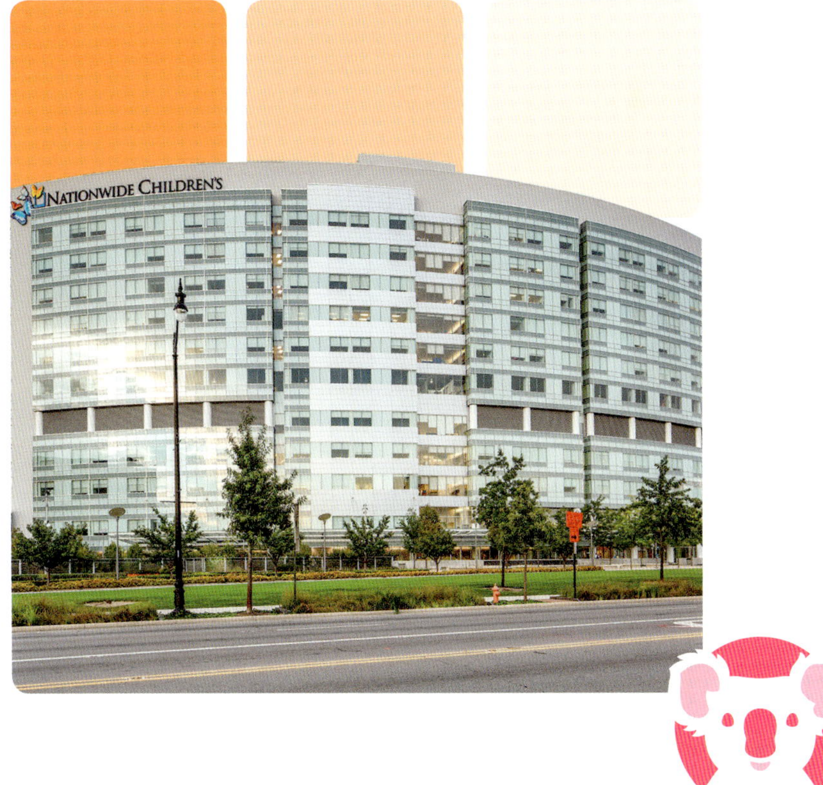

Cody Koala
An Imprint of Pop!
popbooksonline.com

abdobooks.com
Published by Pop!, a division of ABDO, PO Box 398166, Minneapolis, Minnesota 55439.

Printed in the United States of America, North Mankato, Minnesota

052019
092019

THIS BOOK CONTAINS RECYCLED MATERIALS

Cover Photo: SG cityscapes/Alamy
Interior Photos: SG cityscapes/Alamy 1, iStockphoto, 5, 7, 9, 11, 13 (top), 13 (bottom left), 13 (bottom right), 15, 16, 19 (top), 19 (bottom left), 19 (bottom right), 20, 21

Editor: Meg Gaertner
Series Designer: Jake Slavik

Library of Congress Control Number: 2018964600

Publisher's Cataloging-in-Publication Data
Names: Bassier, Emma, author.
Title: Hospitals / by Emma Bassier.
Description: Minneapolis, Minnesota : Pop!, 2020 | Series: Places in my community | Includes online resources and index.
Identifiers: ISBN 9781532163487 (lib. bdg.) | ISBN 9781532164927 (ebook)
Subjects: LCSH: Hospitals--Juvenile literature. | City hospitals--Juvenile literature. | Hospital and community--Juvenile literature. | Hospital patients--Medical care--Juvenile literature.
Classification: DDC 362.11--dc23

Hello! My name is

Cody Koala

Pop open this book and you'll find QR codes like this one, loaded with information, so you can learn even more!

Scan this code* and others like it while you read, or visit the website below to make this book pop.

popbooksonline.com/hospitals

*Scanning QR codes requires a web-enabled smart device with a QR code reader app and a camera.

Table of Contents

Chapter 1

Loud Ambulance

Wee-ooo! Wee-ooo!

An **ambulance** drives by. It has flashing lights. It makes a loud noise. It is taking someone to the hospital.

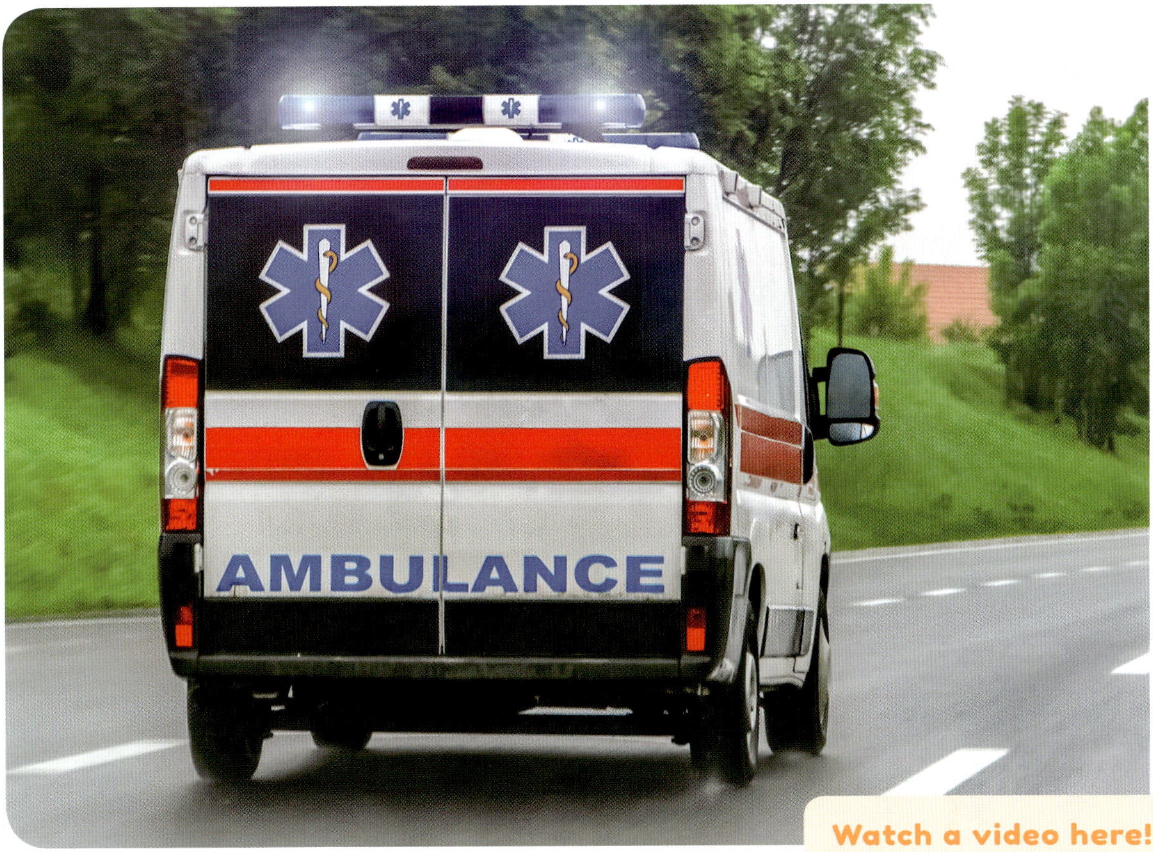

Watch a video here!

Chapter 2

A Place to Heal

A hospital is a place to heal. People go there when they are sick or hurt. They become **patients** at the hospital.

There are more than 5,000 hospitals in the United States.

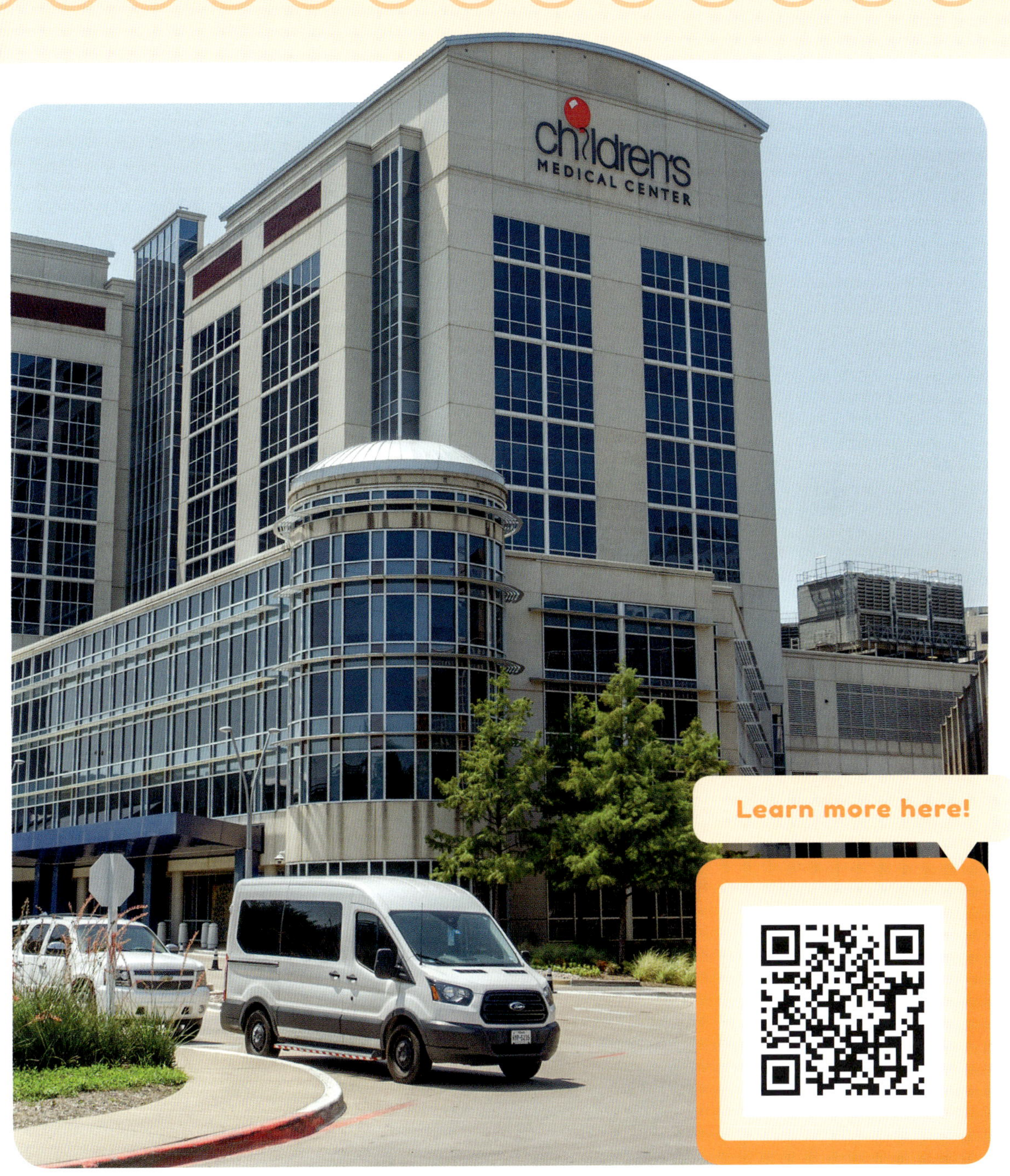

Learn more here!

Patients see **nurses** first. Nurses write down the patient's information. They check the patient's **vital signs**. These signs include temperature and breathing rate.

Another vital sign is how fast the patient's heart is beating.

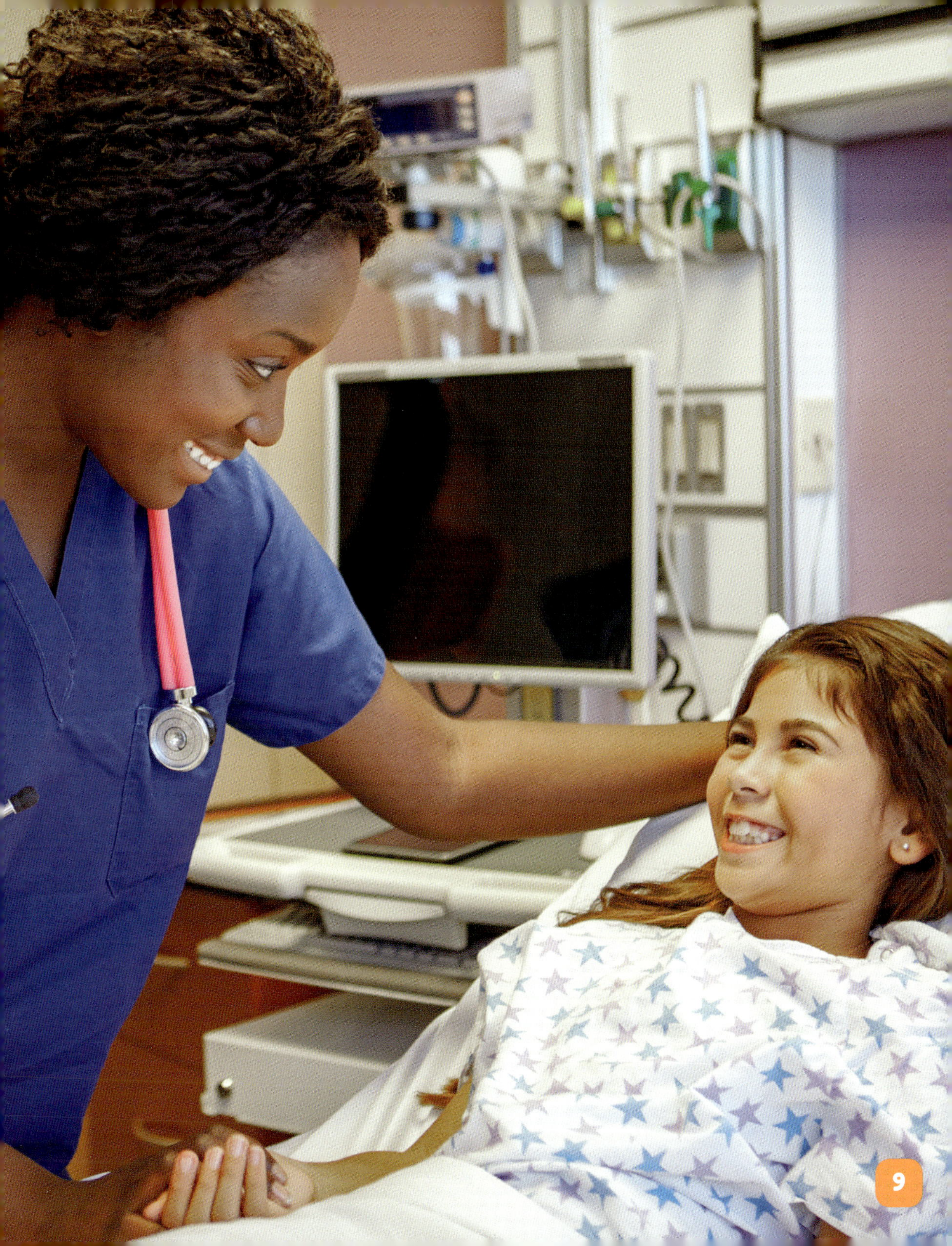

Patients then see a doctor. Doctors say what the problem is. They tell patients what to do about the problem. Patients may need to take medicine. They may need an **operation**.

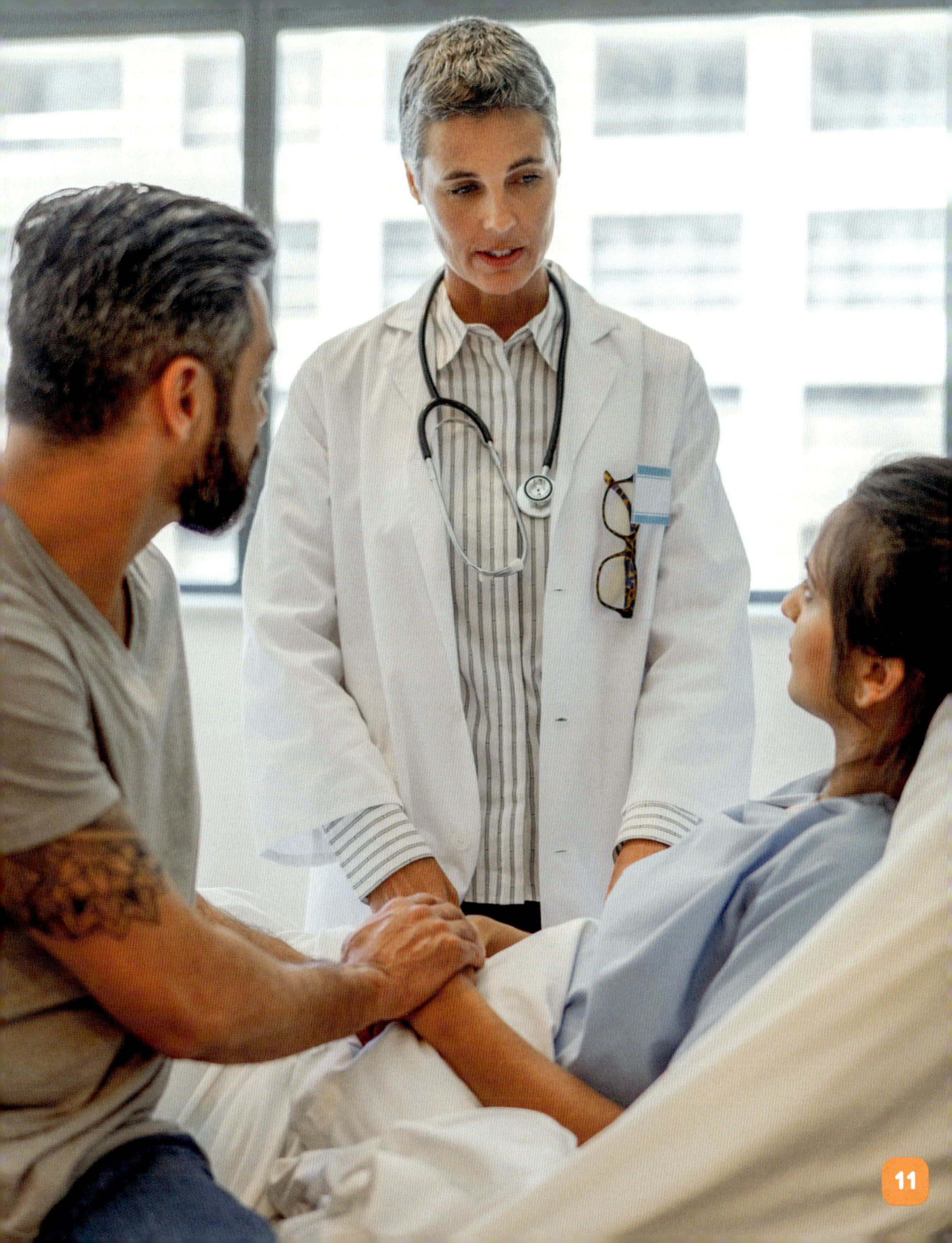

Chapter 3

Inside a Hospital

A hospital has many parts. Many people go to the emergency room first. This place is for people who need help right away.

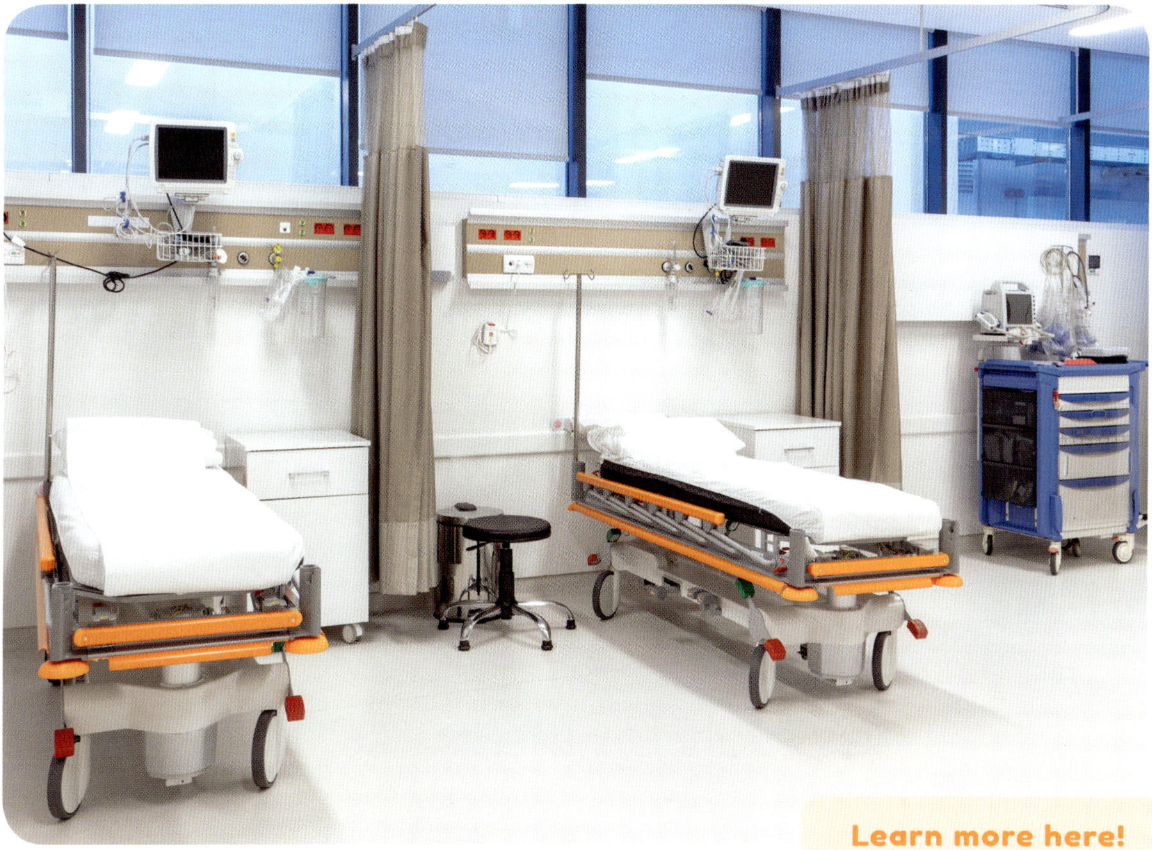

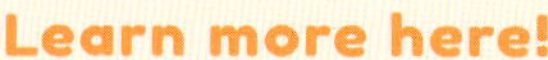
Learn more here!

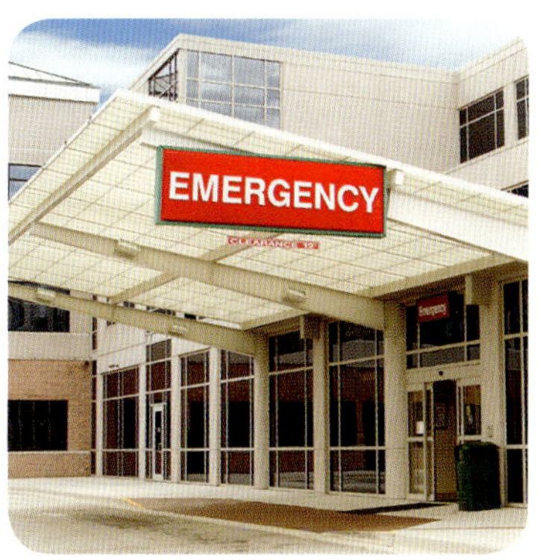
EMERGENCY

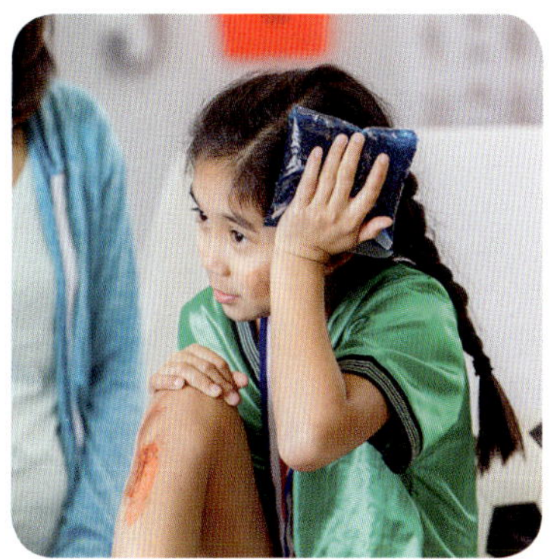

Patients may spend the night at the hospital. They stay in their own room. Or they share with another patient. The room has a bed. It has tools for the **nurse**. It has a curtain. The curtain can be pulled shut to give the patient space.

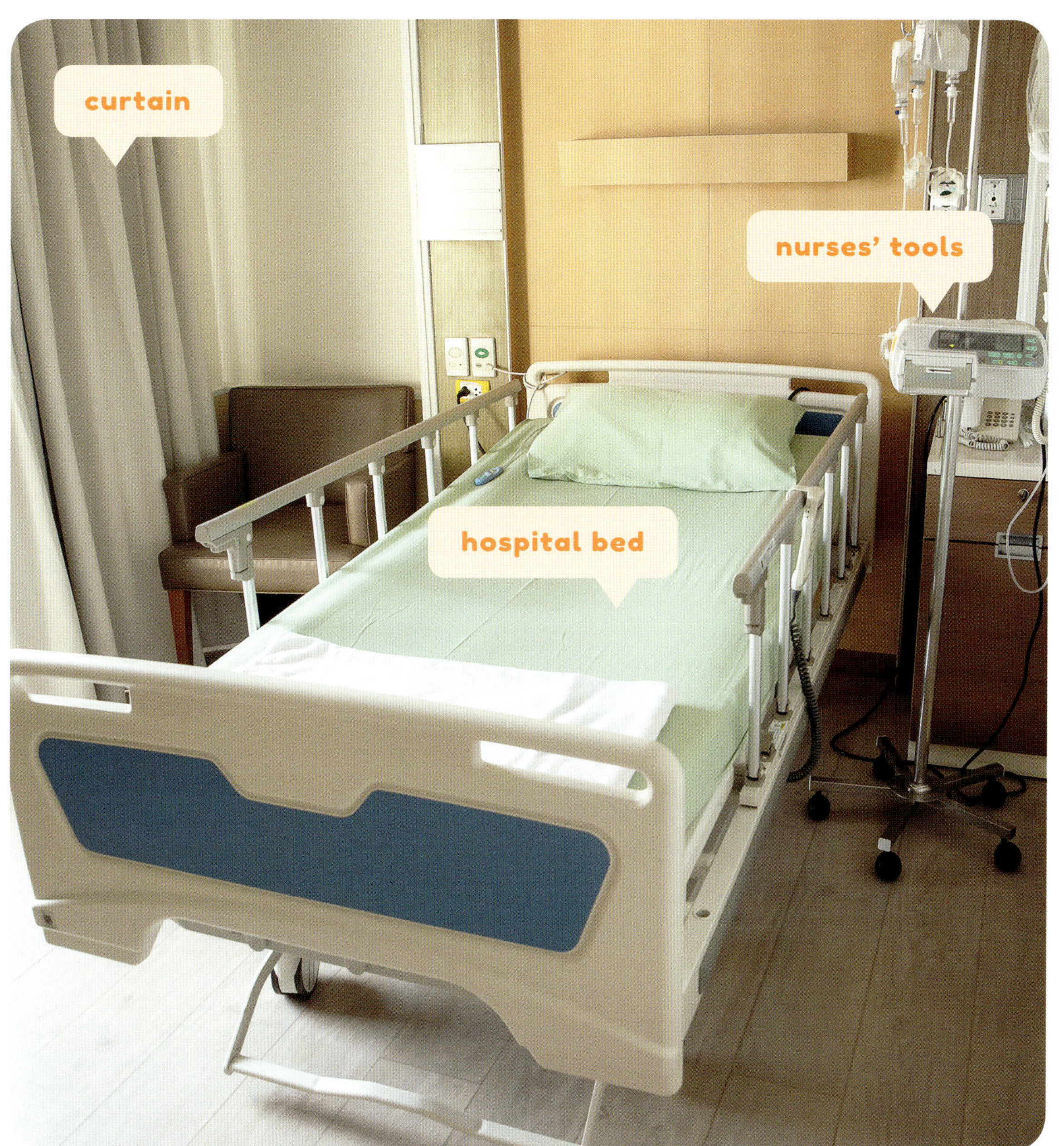
curtain
nurses' tools
hospital bed

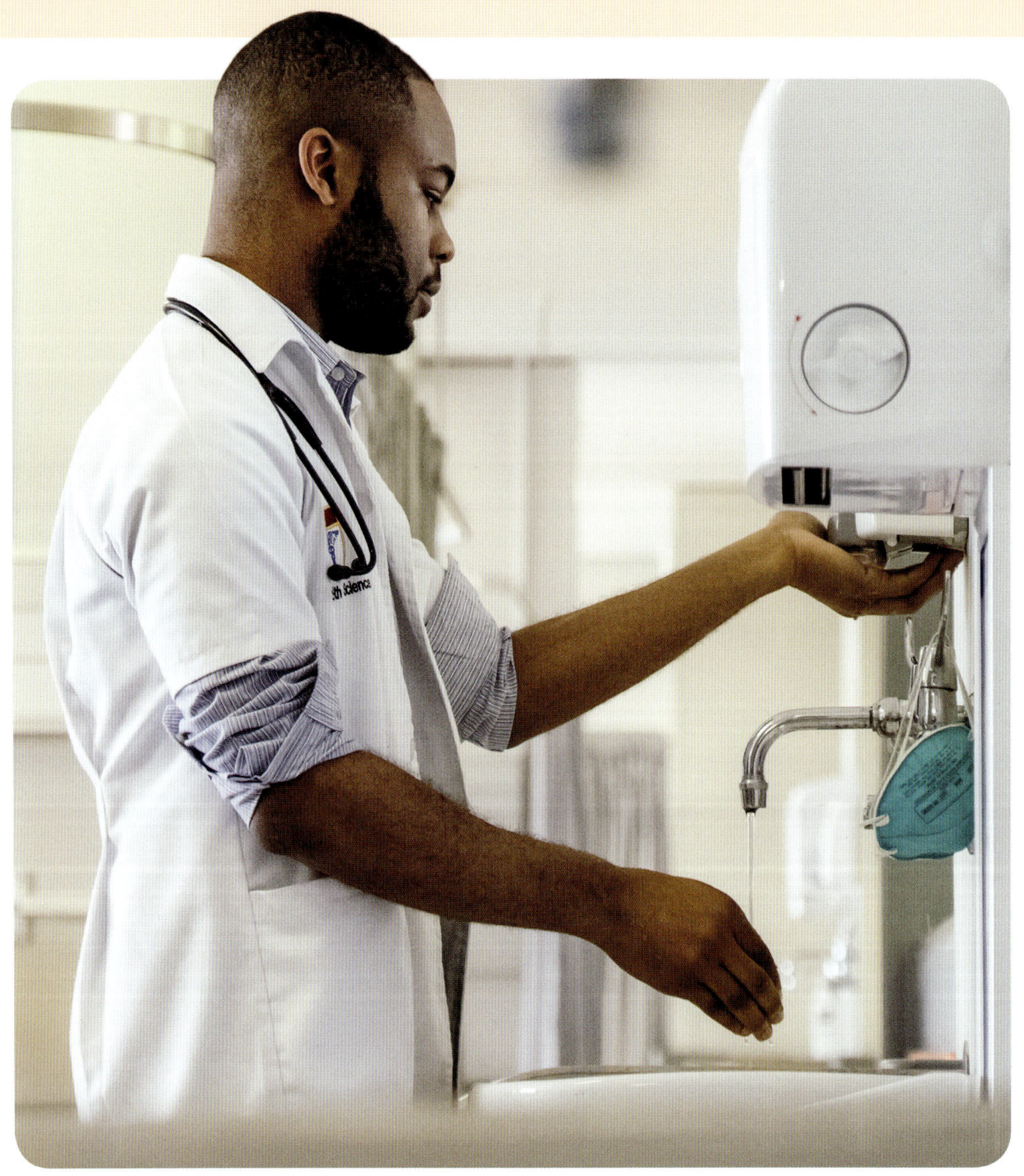

Hospital rooms must stay very clean. Doctors and nurses wash their hands often. They do this so they do not spread germs.

Some doctors focus on the whole body. Others focus on certain body parts.

Chapter 4

Better Life

Hospitals are important to the community. Sometimes people get hurt. Or they do not feel well. They know they can get help at the hospital.

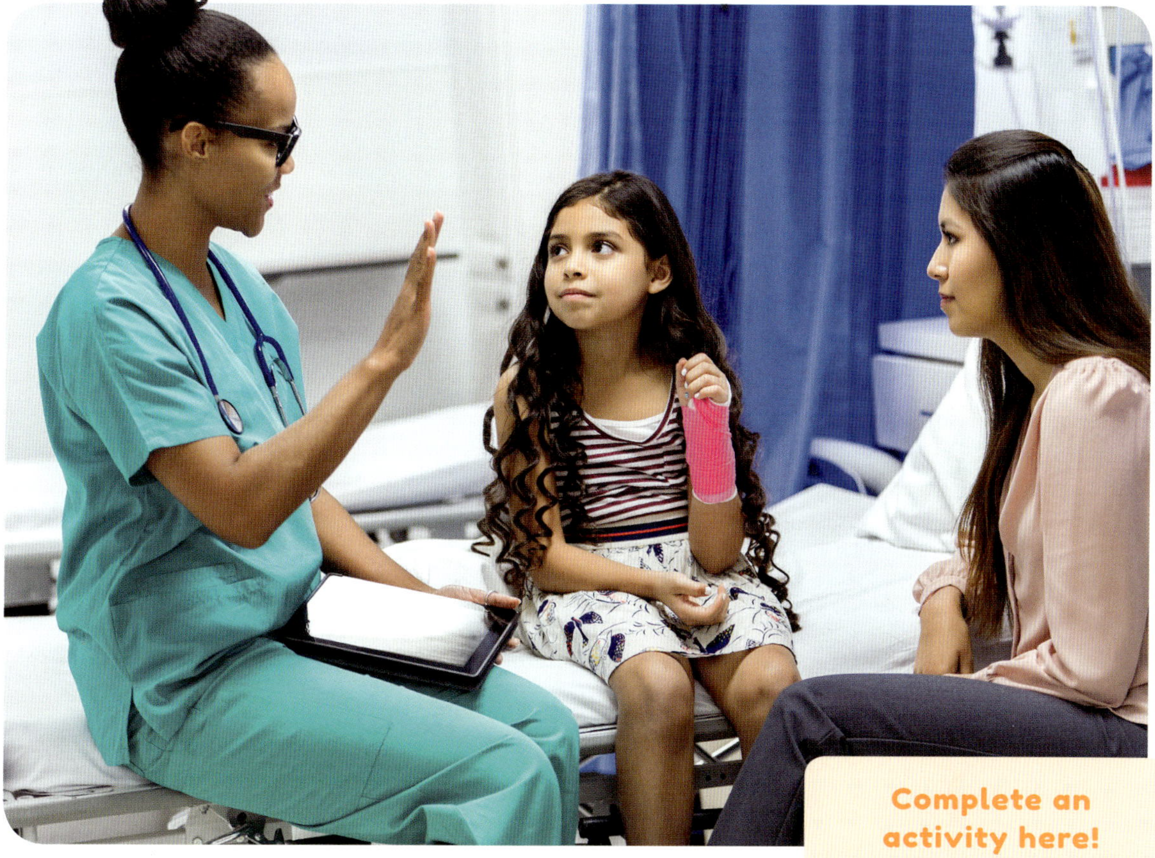

Complete an activity here!

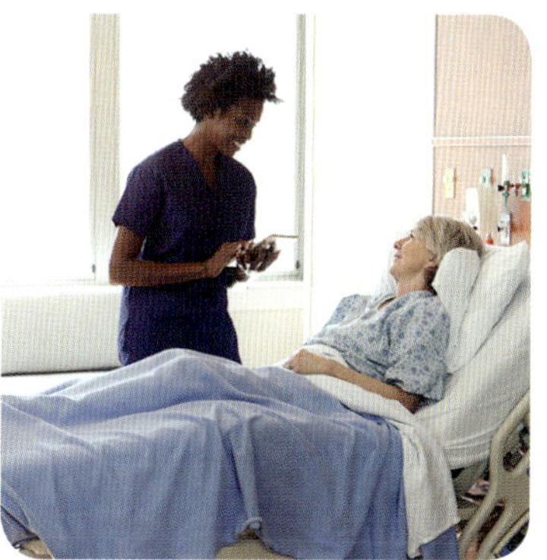

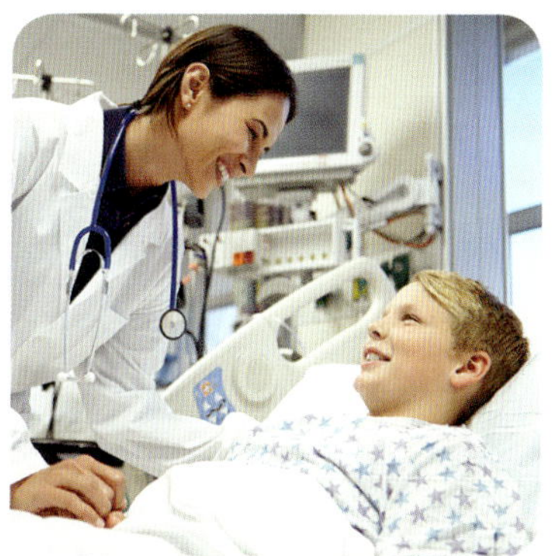

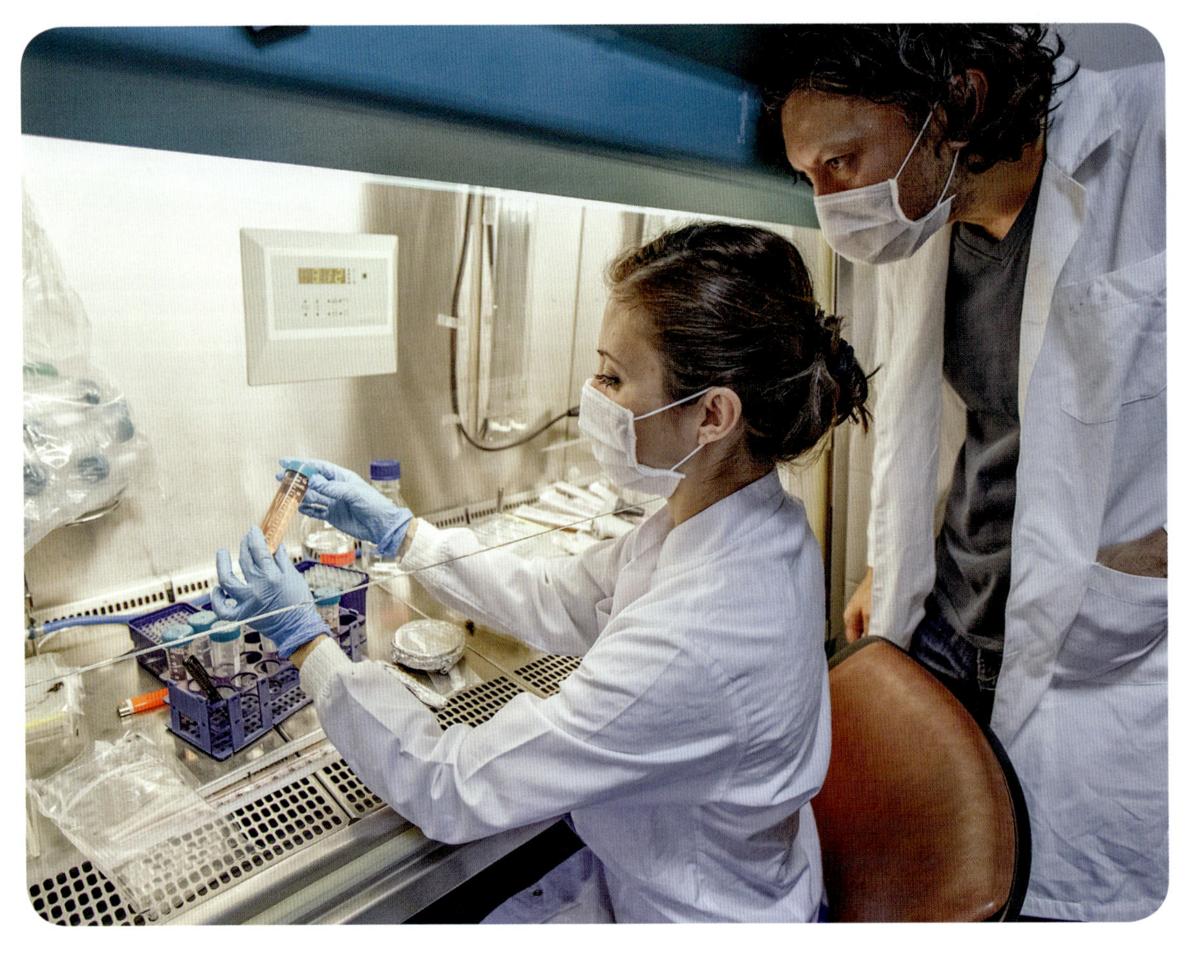

Hospitals also work to find new ways to help people.

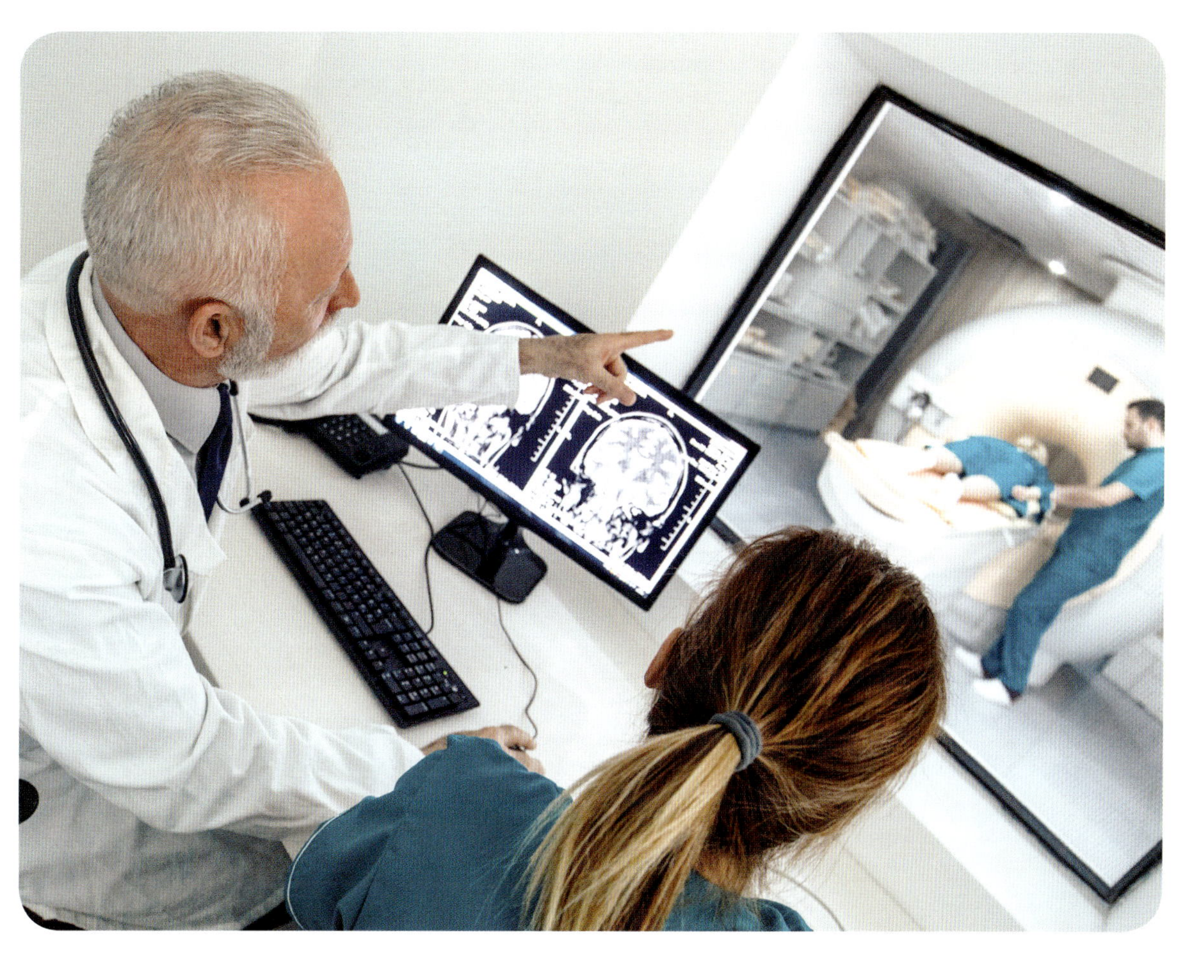

Doctors study health issues.

They find new **treatments**.

Making Connections

Text-to-Self

Have you ever been to the hospital or visited the doctor? What was it like?

Text-to-Text

Have you read other books about hospitals? What did you learn?

Text-to-World

Doctors and nurses help people feel better. Who are some other community helpers?

Glossary

ambulance – a vehicle that gives people medical care while taking them to a hospital.

nurse – a hospital worker who helps patients.

operation – a process in which a doctor cuts into a patient's body to fix or remove a damaged part.

patient – a person receiving medical care.

treatment – medical care given to a patient for an illness or injury.

vital sign – one of the several signs that tell how healthy a person's body is.

Index

Online Resources

popbooksonline.com

Thanks for reading this Cody Koala book!

Scan this code* and others like it in this book, or visit the website below to make this book pop!

popbooksonline.com/hospitals

*Scanning QR codes requires a web-enabled smart device with a QR code reader app and a camera.